How to Slim Down Naturally

Naturally

Harnessing the Power of Plants for Weight Loss

Author

Dr. Lauren D. Goldstein

2023

DISCLAIMER NOTICE

Please keep in mind that the information in this book is strictly for educational purposes. Please consult a licensed specialist before using any of the codes in this book.

Contents

GREEN TEA EXTRACT

INTRODUCTION

Green Tea Extract is highly regarded in the world of herbal remedies for its soothing aroma and its ability to potentially aid in weight management. Green tea has a rich cultural significance that stems from its origins in the Camellia sinensis plant and its use in traditional medicine. There is growing recognition of its ability to improve overall health, particularly in regards to obesity.

BOTANICAL WONDERS

The Camellia sinensis plant, the source of all true teas, is native to East Asia and has been cultivated for centuries for its leaves, which undergo minimal oxidation to produce green tea. This plant's versatility has made it a cornerstone of various cultural practices, from elaborate tea ceremonies in Japan to daily rituals in households worldwide. The leaves' unique biochemical composition, including polyphenols, catechins, and flavonoids, forms the foundation for the therapeutic potential of Green Tea Extract.

ACTIVE COMPOUNDS AND THERAPEUTIC POTENCY

Green Tea Extract possesses a wide array of active compounds that work together to provide numerous health benefits. Catechins, a type of polyphenol, take center stage, with epigallocatechin gallate (EGCG) shining as a standout performer. These compounds, lauded for their antioxidant properties, possess the ability to combat oxidative stress, a key contributor to inflammation and various health issues, including obesity.

The therapeutic potency of Green Tea Extract extends beyond its antioxidant prowess. Research suggests that it may influence various aspects of metabolism, making it a subject of keen interest in the realm of weight management. EGCG, in particular, has been scrutinized for its potential to enhance fat oxidation and contribute to calorie expenditure, potentially aiding individuals in their quest to shed excess weight.

PREPARATION AND DOSAGE

Incorporating Green Tea Extract into one's daily routine can take various forms, with each method offering a delightful and healthful experience. Traditional green tea, prepared by steeping tea leaves in hot water, is a classic choice. For those seeking a more concentrated dose, Green Tea Extract supplements, available in capsules or liquid form, provide a convenient option.

Dosage recommendations may vary based on individual factors, including age, health status, and weight management goals. However, a general guideline is to consume two to three cups of green tea per day, or an equivalent amount in extract form. Starting with a lower dose and gradually increasing can help individuals gauge their tolerance and monitor any potential effects.

SAFETY PRECAUTIONS

While Green Tea Extract is generally considered safe for most individuals when consumed in moderation, certain precautions should be observed. Its moderate caffeine content may affect individuals sensitive to caffeine, leading to potential side effects such as insomnia or increased heart rate. Pregnant or breastfeeding individuals and those with certain medical conditions should exercise caution and consult with a healthcare professional before incorporating Green Tea Extract into their regimen.

INCORPORATING GREEN TEA EXTRACT INTO A HEALTHY LIFESTYLE

In order to fully experience the range of advantages provided by Green Tea Extract for weight management, it is crucial to consider it as a component of a comprehensive approach to overall well-being. Although the potential effects on metabolism and fat oxidation are interesting, it is important to note that Green Tea Extract should not be relied upon as the sole solution. Embracing a holistic approach to your lifestyle, which includes a well-balanced diet, consistent exercise, and proper hydration, is crucial for achieving and sustaining a healthy weight.

Green Tea Extract is incredibly versatile and can easily be incorporated into your daily routine. Whether you prefer it as a soothing warm beverage, a refreshing addition to your smoothies, or as a convenient supplement, it seamlessly fits into your lifestyle. As an addition to other healthy choices, it becomes a valuable partner in the pursuit of overall well-being.

GARCINIA CAMBOGIA

INTRODUCTION

Nestled in the tropical landscapes of Southeast Asia, Garcinia Cambogia emerges as a herbal remedy garnering attention for its purported role in obesity management. Derived from the fruit of the Garcinia gummi-gutta tree, this herbal extract has captured the fascination of those seeking natural solutions for weight-related concerns. As we embark on this exploration, we delve into the botanical wonders, active compounds, scientific research, preparation methods, safety considerations, and the holistic integration of Garcinia Cambogia into a lifestyle aimed at tackling obesity.

BOTANICAL WONDERS

Garcinia Cambogia, also known as Malabar tamarind, brims with botanical wonders that have been harnessed for centuries in traditional culinary practices. The small, pumpkin-shaped fruit, ranging from green to pale yellow in color, houses a wealth of phytochemicals. Native to regions of Indonesia, India, and Southeast Asia, Garcinia Cambogia has found its way into traditional dishes, showcasing both its culinary and potential medicinal applications.

ACTIVE COMPOUNDS AND THERAPEUTIC PROWESS

At the core of Garcinia Cambogia's potential lies hydroxycitric acid (HCA), a citric acid derivative found in the rind of the fruit. HCA is believed to be the key player in the fruit's purported weight management properties. Research suggests that HCA may inhibit an enzyme called citrate lyase, which is involved in the synthesis of fats. Additionally, it is thought to raise serotonin levels, potentially influencing appetite and mood.

The therapeutic prowess of Garcinia Cambogia extends beyond its potential impact on weight management. It has been traditionally used for digestive issues and as a flavoring agent in culinary practices. However, its role in weight management has taken center stage, drawing the attention of researchers and individuals alike.

PREPARATION AND DOSAGE

Adding Garcinia Cambogia to your routine typically includes using dietary supplements, which are commonly found in the form of capsules or liquid extracts. There is some variation in dosage recommendations, but a general guideline suggests a daily intake of 500 to 1500 milligrams of HCA, preferably taken before meals. It is crucial to adhere to the instructions provided for the product and seek guidance from a healthcare professional to establish a suitable dosage that caters to individual requirements.

SAFETY CONSIDERATIONS

While Garcinia Cambogia is generally regarded as safe for short-term use, certain considerations should be taken into account. Common side effects reported in some individuals include digestive issues such as nausea, diarrhea, and stomach discomfort. It's crucial to adhere to recommended dosages, as excessive intake may lead to adverse effects.

Pregnant or breastfeeding individuals, as well as those with pre-existing medical conditions such as diabetes or liver disorders, should exercise caution and seek medical advice before incorporating Garcinia Cambogia into their routine. As with any herbal supplement, it is advisable to consult with a healthcare professional to assess potential interactions with medications and overall suitability for individual health profiles.

HOLISTIC INTEGRATION INTO LIFESTYLE

Garcinia Cambogia, when considered as part of a holistic approach to obesity management, becomes one element in a larger tapestry of healthy living. It is not a magic solution but rather a potential ally in the journey towards weight management. Adopting a lifestyle that includes a balanced diet, regular physical activity, and mindful eating remains foundational to achieving sustainable and holistic well-being.

The inclusion of Garcinia Cambogia in dietary practices can be complemented by making healthful choices in other aspects of life. Engaging in regular exercise, staying hydrated, and prioritizing sleep are integral components of a lifestyle aimed at addressing obesity and fostering overall health.

GINGER

INTRODUCTION

Ginger (Zingiber officinale) possesses a unique and delightful aroma and taste that sets it apart from other plants. Ginger has been highly regarded in traditional medicine for centuries due to its numerous health benefits, extending beyond its culinary appeal. This unique plant, with its intricate tangled roots, shows potential in the field of weight management. As we delve into the wonders of ginger, its powerful compounds, scientific studies, culinary uses, and how it can be incorporated into a healthy lifestyle, we discover it's potential to support those striving to address obesity.

BOTANICAL MARVELS

Ginger, a member of the Zingiberaceae family, is a tropical plant native to Southeast Asia. Its rhizomes, often referred to as ginger roots, boast a pungent and slightly sweet flavor, adding depth to both savory and sweet dishes. Beyond its culinary applications, ginger has been revered for its medicinal properties across diverse cultures. The plant's knotted rhizomes, often used fresh, dried, or as an extract, house a complex array of bioactive compounds that contribute to its therapeutic potential.

ACTIVE COMPOUNDS AND THERAPEUTIC PROWESS

At the heart of ginger's therapeutic prowess lie bioactive compounds such as gingerol, shogaol, and paradol. These compounds, belonging to the family of phenolic compounds, confer anti-inflammatory, antioxidant, and antiemetic properties to ginger.

Gingerol, the primary bioactive compound, is lauded for its potent antioxidant effects. Antioxidants play a crucial role in neutralizing free radicals, which contribute to oxidative stress and inflammation—factors intricately linked to obesity-related complications. Moreover, gingerol exhibits anti-inflammatory effects that may impact the inflammatory pathways associated with obesity.

PREPARATION AND CULINARY APPLICATIONS

Incorporating ginger into one's dietary regimen is not only healthful but also a culinary delight. Fresh ginger can be grated, sliced, or minced and added to a variety of dishes, ranging from stir-fries to teas and desserts. Dried ginger powder is a versatile option, seamlessly integrating into spice blends and baked goods.

For those seeking a concentrated dose of ginger, ginger supplements, including capsules and extracts, offer a convenient option. However, the joy of experiencing ginger's therapeutic benefits through culinary exploration adds an extra layer of pleasure to its incorporation into daily life.

HOLISTIC INTEGRATION INTO A HEALTHFUL LIFESTYLE

Ginger's potential as an herbal remedy for obesity unfolds most effectively when viewed as part of a comprehensive strategy for well-being. While the scientific findings provide valuable insights, ginger is not a standalone solution. Rather, it thrives in synergy with other healthful practices.

Adopting a lifestyle that encompasses a balanced diet rich in whole foods, regular physical activity, and mindful eating lays the groundwork for effective obesity management. Ginger, with its array of bioactive compounds, becomes a flavorful and healthful ally in this holistic approach.

SAFETY CONSIDERATIONS

Ginger is generally considered safe for most individuals when consumed in moderate amounts. However, some individuals may experience mild side effects such as heartburn or digestive discomfort. Pregnant or breastfeeding individuals and those with certain medical conditions, such as gallstones or bleeding disorders, should exercise caution and seek guidance from healthcare professionals before incorporating ginger into their routine.

CAYENNE PEPPER

INTRODUCTION

In the colorful realm of herbal remedies, cayenne pepper (Capsicum annuum) stands out as a bold contender, both in terms of its spicy flavor and the potential health benefits it offers. Famous for its fiery flavor, this chili pepper relative is not just a tasty treat but has also gained recognition for its possible contribution to weight management. As we explore the fascinating world of cayenne pepper, we delve into its active compounds, scientific research, culinary uses, and its potential to promote wellness in the fight against obesity.

BOTANICAL INTRICACIES

Cayenne pepper, derived from dried and ground chili peppers, belongs to the Capsicum annuum species. The vibrant red hue of cayenne peppers is indicative of the presence of capsaicinoids, the bioactive compounds responsible for their spicy flavor and potential health-promoting effects. Native to Central and South America, cayenne pepper has traversed culinary and medicinal landscapes, leaving its mark on diverse cultures.

ACTIVE COMPOUNDS AND THERAPEUTIC IGNITION

At the heart of cayenne pepper's therapeutic potential lies capsaicin, the primary capsaicinoid responsible for its heat. Capsaicin engages with receptors in the body, particularly the transient receptor potential vanilloid I (TRPVI), triggering a cascade of physiological responses. This interaction is not only responsible for the fiery sensation experienced when consuming cayenne pepper but also for the potential health benefits associated with its consumption.

Research has unveiled capsaicin's multifaceted impact, ranging from its role in pain modulation to its potential influence on metabolic processes. In the context of obesity management, capsaicin is believed to contribute to increased calorie expenditure and fat oxidation, making cayenne pepper a subject of interest in the pursuit of weight-related goals.

PREPARATION AND CULINARY APPLICATIONS

Incorporating cayenne pepper into one's culinary repertoire can be both a healthful and flavorful endeavor. The spice can be used in various forms, including dried powder, flakes, or as a fresh pepper.

Its versatile nature allows for seamless integration into an array of dishes, from soups and stews to sauces and marinades.

For those seeking a concentrated dose of capsaicin, cayenne pepper supplements, available in capsule form, offer a convenient option. However, the joy of experiencing cayenne pepper's potential benefits through culinary exploration adds an extra layer of pleasure to its incorporation into daily life.

HOLISTIC INTEGRATION INTO A HEALTHFUL LIFESTYLE

Cayenne pepper's potential as an herbal remedy for obesity unfolds most effectively when viewed as part of a comprehensive strategy for well-being. While scientific findings provide valuable insights, cayenne pepper is not a standalone solution. Rather, it thrives in synergy with other healthful practices.

A balanced diet rich in whole foods, regular physical activity, and mindful eating lays the groundwork for effective obesity management. Cayenne pepper, with its capsaicin content, becomes a flavorful and healthful ally in this holistic approach.

SAFETY CONSIDERATIONS

While cayenne pepper is generally considered safe for most individuals when consumed in moderation, certain considerations should be taken into account. The spice's heat may pose challenges for individuals with sensitive stomachs or conditions such as acid reflux. Gradual incorporation and monitoring of tolerance are advisable.

Pregnant or breastfeeding individuals and those with certain medical conditions, such as gastrointestinal disorders or allergies, should exercise caution and seek guidance from healthcare professionals before incorporating cayenne pepper into their routine.

CINNAMON

INTRODUCTION

Cinnamon, also known as Cinnamomum verum, is a truly delightful and flavorful spice that is highly cherished for its captivating aroma and potential benefits for overall wellness. Cinnamon has become increasingly recognized for its potential health benefits, particularly in relation to weight management. It is not only a popular spice in the kitchen but also has gained attention for its potential effects on overall health. As we explore the intriguing realm of cinnamon, we will discover its potent compounds, analyze scientific research, delve into its culinary applications, and contemplate its potential in supporting a comprehensive approach to achieving weight-related objectives.

BOTANICAL WONDERS

Cinnamon, derived from the inner bark of Cinnamomum verum trees, boasts a rich history intertwined with ancient trade routes and cultural practices. Native to Sri Lanka and other parts of Southeast Asia, cinnamon has traversed time and continents, leaving its aromatic imprint on diverse cuisines and traditional medicines. The spice's distinctive sweet and spicy flavor is owed to a complex profile of active compounds, making cinnamon not only a culinary delight but also a potential herbal ally.

ACTIVE COMPOUNDS AND THERAPEUTIC AROMA

At the heart of cinnamon's therapeutic potential lie key compounds, including cinnamaldehyde, cinnamic acid, and cinnamate. These compounds contribute not only to the spice's delightful aroma and flavor but also to its potential health-promoting effects.

Cinnamaldehyde, the primary component responsible for cinnamon's characteristic flavor, is also attributed with antioxidant and anti-inflammatory properties. Antioxidants play a crucial role in neutralizing free radicals, which contribute to oxidative stress and inflammation—factors intricately linked to obesity-related complications.

PREPARATION AND CULINARY APPLICATIONS

Incorporating cinnamon into one's culinary repertoire is not only a healthful endeavor but also a flavorful one. The spice can be used in various forms, including ground cinnamon, cinnamon sticks, or as an essential oil. Its versatility allows for seamless integration into an array of dishes, from breakfast favorites like oatmeal and yogurt to savory stews and baked goods.

For those seeking a concentrated dose of cinnamon's active compounds, cinnamon supplements, available in capsule form, offer a convenient option. However, the joy of experiencing cinnamon's potential benefits through culinary exploration adds an extra layer of pleasure to its incorporation into daily life.

HOLISTIC INTEGRATION INTO A HEALTHFUL LIFESTYLE

Cinnamon's potential as an herbal remedy for obesity unfolds most effectively when viewed as part of a comprehensive strategy for well-being. While scientific findings provide valuable insights, cinnamon is not a standalone solution. Rather, it thrives in synergy with other healthful practices.

A balanced diet rich in whole foods, regular physical activity, and mindful eating lays the groundwork for effective obesity management. Cinnamon, with its bioactive compounds, becomes a flavorful and healthful ally in this holistic approach.

SAFETY CONSIDERATIONS

Cinnamon is generally considered safe for most individuals when consumed in moderation. However, certain considerations should be taken into account, particularly for individuals with sensitivity or allergies to cinnamon. Cassia cinnamon, a common variety, contains coumarin, a compound that may be harmful in high doses. Ceylon cinnamon, a milder variety, is considered a safer alternative.

Pregnant or breastfeeding individuals and those with certain medical conditions, such as liver disorders, should exercise caution and seek guidance from healthcare professionals before incorporating cinnamon into their routine.

DANDELION

INTRODUCTION

When it comes to natural healing, one particular plant stands out - dandelion (Taraxacum officinale). This humble botanical ally is renowned for its numerous health benefits and is often used in herbal remedies. Often overlooked as an unwanted plant, the dandelion has a fascinating background in ancient healing practices and culinary customs. In addition to its lovely yellow flowers, dandelion shows potential as a herbal remedy for those seeking to manage their weight. Through this exploration, we will delve into the fascinating world of dandelion, exploring its botanical properties, active compounds, scientific studies, culinary uses, and its potential as a holistic aid in combating obesity.

BOTANICAL WONDERS

Dandelion, with its bright yellow flowers and distinctive serrated leaves, is a familiar sight in gardens and meadows across the globe. Despite its reputation as a weed, this perennial herb has been valued for centuries in various cultural traditions for its medicinal properties. Native to Europe and Asia, dandelion has found its way into diverse herbal practices, gaining recognition for its diuretic, detoxifying, and potentially weight-modulating effects.

ACTIVE COMPOUNDS AND THERAPEUTIC MARVELS

The therapeutic potency of dandelion lies in its rich array of bioactive compounds, including flavonoids, sesquiterpene lactones, and taraxasterol. These compounds contribute to dandelion's diuretic properties, supporting the elimination of excess fluids and waste from the body.

Flavonoids, powerful antioxidants found in dandelion, play a crucial role in neutralizing free radicals, combating oxidative stress, and contributing to overall cellular health. Sesquiterpene lactones are compounds with anti-inflammatory properties, potentially influencing processes related to obesity and metabolic health. Taraxasterol, another component of dandelion, has been studied for its potential role in modulating lipid metabolism.

PREPARATION AND CULINARY APPLICATIONS

Incorporating dandelion into one's diet can take various forms, with both the leaves and roots being utilized. Dandelion leaves can be harvested and added to salads, sautéed as a side dish, or used in smoothies. The roots are often dried and roasted to make a caffeine-free dandelion coffee alternative.

Dandelion tea, made from the leaves or roots, is a popular and convenient way to enjoy the herb's potential benefits. Additionally, dandelion supplements, available in various forms such as capsules or tinctures, offer a concentrated and accessible option for those seeking a more targeted approach.

HOLISTIC INTEGRATION INTO A HEALTHFUL LIFESTYLE

Dandelion's potential as an herbal remedy for obesity unfolds most effectively when viewed as part of a comprehensive strategy for well-being. While research provides insights into specific aspects of dandelion's potential impact on weight-related factors, it is crucial to integrate its consumption into a broader context of healthful living.

A balanced and nutrient-dense diet, regular physical activity, and mindful eating practices remain foundational to effective weight management. Dandelion, with its diuretic and potential detoxifying effects, can complement these lifestyle choices by supporting the body's natural processes.

SAFETY CONSIDERATIONS

Dandelion is generally regarded as safe for most individuals when consumed in moderation. However, there are considerations to keep in mind. Individuals allergic to plants in the Asteraceae family, such as ragweed or marigolds, may experience allergic reactions to dandelion. Additionally, those with certain medical conditions, such as gallstones or kidney issues, should exercise caution and consult with healthcare professionals before incorporating dandelion into their routine.

FENUGREEK

INTRODUCTION

When it comes to natural remedies, fenugreek (Trigonella foenum-graecum) stands out as a powerful botanical ally that is highly regarded for its wide range of health benefits and uses in cooking. Hailing from the Mediterranean region, fenugreek has made its way through various cultures and traditions, making an impact in both traditional medicine and delicious culinary dishes. In addition to its fragrant seeds and unique bitter flavor, fenugreek shows potential as a natural remedy in the quest for managing obesity. Through this extensive investigation, we explore the fascinating world of fenugreek, examining its botanical properties, powerful compounds, scientific studies, culinary uses, and its potential to support a holistic approach to combatting obesity.

BOTANICAL WONDERS

Fenugreek, with its delicate leaves and small, golden-brown seeds, is a member of the Fabaceae family. Native to the Mediterranean region, it has been cultivated for centuries for its culinary and medicinal properties. Fenugreek leaves are commonly used as a leafy green in various cuisines, while the seeds are prized for their aromatic and slightly bitter taste. The plant's botanical wonders lie in its rich nutrient profile, which includes proteins, dietary fibers, vitamins, and minerals.

ACTIVE COMPOUNDS AND THERAPEUTIC MARVELS

The therapeutic potential of fenugreek is attributed to its diverse array of bioactive compounds, including saponins, flavonoids, alkaloids, and fibers. Notably, fenugreek seeds contain a unique group of compounds called trigonelline, which has been studied for its potential health benefits.

Saponins, found abundantly in fenugreek, exhibit anti-inflammatory and antioxidant properties. These compounds contribute to fenugreek's potential role in addressing oxidative stress and inflammation, factors intricately linked to obesity-related complications.

PREPARATION AND CULINARY APPLICATIONS

Incorporating fenugreek into culinary practices is not only a healthful endeavor but also a flavorful one. Fenugreek seeds can be used whole or ground and are often added to spice blends, curries, and pickles. Fenugreek leaves, known as methi in Indian cuisine, add a distinctive flavor to dishes such as curries and flatbreads.

Fenugreek supplements, including capsules, powders, or extracts, offer a convenient option for those seeking a concentrated dose of its bioactive compounds. However, the joy of experiencing fenugreek's potential benefits through culinary exploration adds an extra layer of pleasure to its incorporation into daily life.

HOLISTIC INTEGRATION INTO A HEALTHFUL LIFESTYLE

Fenugreek's potential as an herbal remedy for obesity unfolds most effectively when viewed as part of a comprehensive strategy for well-being. While scientific findings provide valuable insights, fenugreek is not a standalone solution. Rather, it thrives in synergy with other healthful practices.

A balanced and nutrient-dense diet, regular physical activity, and mindful eating practices remain foundational to effective weight management. Fenugreek, with its unique combination of fibers, proteins, and bioactive compounds, can complement these lifestyle choices by supporting metabolic health and contributing to satiety.

SAFETY CONSIDERATIONS

Fenugreek is generally considered safe for most individuals when consumed in moderate amounts. However, certain considerations should be taken into account. Some individuals may experience allergic reactions to fenugreek, particularly those with allergies to other plants in the Fabaceae family, such as peanuts or chickpeas.

Pregnant or breastfeeding individuals should exercise caution, as fenugreek has been traditionally used to stimulate lactation, and its safety during pregnancy and breastfeeding is not well-established. Additionally, individuals with certain medical conditions, such as diabetes or hypoglycemia, should monitor their blood sugar levels, as fenugreek may impact blood glucose regulation.

TURMERIC

INTRODUCTION

Turmeric, known as Curcuma longa, is a remarkable spice with a rich history in both traditional medicine and culinary practices. Hailing from South Asia, turmeric has surpassed borders to become a widely acclaimed spice around the world. In addition to its delicious flavor, turmeric has been acknowledged for its potential to promote good health, particularly in relation to managing weight. In this exploration, we explore the fascinating world of turmeric, examining its botanical properties, powerful compounds, extensive scientific research, versatile culinary uses, and its potential to support holistic well-being in the fight against obesity.

BOTANICAL WONDERS

Turmeric, a member of the ginger family, is a perennial plant known for its vibrant golden-yellow rhizomes. Native to South Asia, turmeric has been a staple in traditional Ayurvedic medicine for centuries. The rhizomes, when harvested, dried, and ground, yield the distinctive spice that imparts both color and flavor to a myriad of dishes. Turmeric's botanical wonders are encapsulated in its active compound, curcumin, which gives it not only its characteristic hue but also its potential health-promoting properties.

ACTIVE COMPOUNDS AND THERAPEUTIC MARVELS

The primary active compound in turmeric, curcumin, is a polyphenol with potent antioxidant and anti-inflammatory properties. These properties make curcumin a key player in addressing oxidative stress and inflammation, both of which are intricately linked to obesity and its associated complications.

Beyond curcumin, turmeric contains other bioactive compounds, such as turmerones and curcuminoids, each contributing to its holistic therapeutic potential. Turmerones, for instance, have been studied for their potential neuroprotective and anti-inflammatory effects.

PREPARATION AND CULINARY APPLICATIONS

Incorporating turmeric into daily culinary practices is not only a healthful endeavor but also a flavorful one. Turmeric can be used in various forms, including fresh rhizomes, dried powder, or as an essential oil. Its versatility allows for seamless integration into an array of dishes, from curries and stews to soups, rice, and even beverages like golden milk.

Turmeric supplements, available in capsules or extracts, offer a concentrated and convenient option for those seeking a higher dosage of curcumin. However, the joy of experiencing turmeric's potential benefits through culinary exploration adds an extra layer of pleasure to its incorporation into daily life.

HOLISTIC INTEGRATION INTO A HEALTHFUL LIFESTYLE

Turmeric's potential as an herbal remedy for obesity unfolds most effectively when viewed as part of a comprehensive strategy for well-being. While scientific findings provide valuable insights, turmeric is not a standalone solution. Rather, it thrives in synergy with other healthful practices.

A balanced and nutrient-dense diet, regular physical activity, and mindful eating practices remain foundational to effective weight management. Turmeric, with its anti-inflammatory, antioxidant, and potential metabolism-modulating effects, can complement these lifestyle choices by supporting the body's natural processes.

SAFETY CONSIDERATIONS

Turmeric is generally considered safe for most individuals when consumed in moderation. However, some considerations should be taken into account. Curcumin, the active compound in turmeric, may interact with certain medications, such as blood thinners and anticoagulants, so individuals taking these medications should consult with healthcare professionals.

Additionally, individuals with gallbladder issues or those prone to kidney stones should exercise caution, as high doses of turmeric may exacerbate these conditions. Pregnant or breastfeeding individuals should also consult with healthcare professionals before incorporating turmeric into their routine.

ALOE VERA

INTRODUCTION

Aloe Vera, also known as Aloe barbadensis miller, is highly regarded for its wide range of healing properties. Hailing from the arid regions of North Africa, Aloe Vera has surpassed geographical boundaries to become a worldwide emblem of well-being. Although often associated with its external uses, this versatile plant has undiscovered possibilities in treating internal health issues, such as its potential in managing obesity. Join us on a deep dive into the world of Aloe Vera, where we'll explore its botanical complexities, powerful compounds, extensive scientific studies, versatile culinary uses, and its potential as a natural aid in the fight against obesity.

BOTANICAL INTRICACIES

Aloe Vera, belonging to the succulent family, is characterized by its fleshy green leaves that house a gel-like substance. This gel, when extracted, contains a myriad of bioactive compounds that contribute to Aloe Vera's healing prowess. Native to arid climates, Aloe Vera has been treasured for centuries in various traditional medicinal practices, with its uses ranging from skin ailments to internal wellness. The plant's ability to thrive in challenging conditions reflects its resilience and adaptability, qualities that extend to its potential in supporting overall health.

ACTIVE COMPOUNDS AND THERAPEUTIC POTENCY

The therapeutic potency of Aloe Vera lies in its rich array of bioactive compounds, including polysaccharides, anthraquinones, amino acids, vitamins, and minerals. These compounds work synergistically to offer a spectrum of health benefits, both internally and externally.

Polysaccharides, particularly acemannan, are recognized for their immune-modulating properties and potential role in supporting gastrointestinal health. Anthraquinones, known for their laxative effects, contribute to Aloe Vera's historical use in addressing digestive concerns. Amino acids, essential building blocks of proteins, play a role in cellular repair and regeneration. Combined with vitamins and minerals, Aloe Vera becomes a holistic powerhouse, offering a range of nutrients crucial for overall well-being.

PREPARATION AND CULINARY APPLICATIONS

Incorporating Aloe Vera into daily life can take various forms, with Aloe Vera gel being a central component. The gel can be extracted from the leaves and added to smoothies, juices, or incorporated into recipes for a refreshing twist. Aloe Vera supplements, available in various forms such as capsules or extracts, offer a concentrated option for those seeking a higher dosage of its bioactive compounds.

While Aloe Vera gel is commonly associated with topical applications, it is essential to note that not all Aloe Vera products are suitable for internal consumption. Products specifically labeled for internal use should be chosen to ensure safety and efficacy. Additionally, Aloe Vera should be consumed in moderation, as excessive intake may lead to adverse effects.

HOLISTIC INTEGRATION INTO A HEALTHFUL LIFESTYLE

Aloe Vera's potential as an herbal remedy for obesity unfolds most effectively when viewed as part of a comprehensive strategy for well-being. While scientific findings provide valuable insights, Aloe Vera is not a standalone solution. Rather, it thrives in synergy with other healthful practices.

A balanced and nutrient-dense diet, regular physical activity, and mindful eating practices remain foundational to effective weight management. Aloe Vera, with its potential digestive and anti-inflammatory effects, can complement these lifestyle choices by supporting gut health and mitigating inflammation.

SAFETY CONSIDERATIONS

While Aloe Vera is generally safe for topical use and internal consumption when used appropriately, certain considerations should be taken into account. Aloe latex, a substance derived from the inner leaf skin, contains compounds with laxative effects (anthraquinones) and should be used with caution. Prolonged or excessive consumption of Aloe latex may lead to electrolyte imbalances and digestive issues.

It is crucial to choose Aloe Vera products specifically labeled for internal use and consult with healthcare professionals before incorporating Aloe Vera into the routine, especially for individuals with existing medical conditions or those taking medications.

LICORICE ROOT

INTRODUCTION

In the vast landscape of herbal remedies, Licorice Root (Glycyrrhiza glabra) emerges as a sweet and potent ally, celebrated for its distinctive flavor and diverse health benefits. Originating from the Mediterranean and Asia, licorice has traversed cultures and traditions, leaving its mark not only on confectioneries but also in traditional medicinal practices. Beyond its role as a sweetener, licorice root holds promise as an herbal remedy in the pursuit of obesity management. In this in-depth exploration, we navigate through the botanical nuances, active compounds, scientific research, culinary applications, and holistic integration of licorice root, unraveling its potential as a natural ally in the battle against obesity.

BOTANICAL NUANCES

Licorice, derived from the roots of Glycyrrhiza glabra, is a perennial herbaceous plant known for its sweet taste and distinctive aroma. The plant's root system is where the medicinal properties lie, and it has been utilized for centuries in various traditional healing systems, including Ayurveda and Traditional Chinese Medicine. Licorice's botanical nuances include compound roots with a characteristic sweet flavor, making it a popular natural sweetener. The root's adaptability and resilience have allowed it to become a global botanical treasure, finding its way into culinary creations, herbal remedies, and even modern medicine.

ACTIVE COMPOUNDS AND THERAPEUTIC POTENTIAL

The therapeutic potential of licorice root is attributed to a complex array of bioactive compounds, with glycyrrhizin being the most notable. Glycyrrhizin, a triterpene glycoside, is responsible for licorice's intense sweetness and is a key player in its potential health benefits. Beyond glycyrrhizin, licorice root contains flavonoids, coumarins, and other compounds that contribute to its diverse pharmacological actions.

Glycyrrhizin has been studied for its anti-inflammatory, antioxidant, and immunomodulatory properties. These properties make licorice root a potential candidate for addressing conditions associated with inflammation, including those linked to obesity.

PREPARATION AND CULINARY APPLICATIONS

Incorporating licorice root into culinary practices and daily life can take various forms, with licorice root extract, powder, or whole roots being utilized. Licorice root tea, made by infusing the dried root in hot water, is a popular and convenient way to enjoy its potential benefits. Additionally, licorice supplements, available in various forms such as capsules or tinctures, offer a concentrated and accessible option for those seeking a more targeted approach.

Licorice root's sweet flavor makes it a versatile ingredient in both sweet and savory dishes. It is used in traditional candies, desserts, and beverages, as well as in savory dishes like stews and soups. However, it's crucial to use licorice root in moderation, as excessive consumption may lead to potential side effects associated with glycyrrhizin.

HOLISTIC INTEGRATION INTO A HEALTHFUL LIFESTYLE

Licorice root's potential as an herbal remedy for obesity unfolds most effectively when viewed as part of a comprehensive strategy for well-being. While scientific findings provide valuable insights, licorice root is not a standalone solution. Rather, it thrives in synergy with other healthful practices.

A balanced and nutrient-dense diet, regular physical activity, and mindful eating practices remain foundational to effective weight management. Licorice root, with its potential anti-inflammatory, antioxidant, and appetite-regulating effects, can complement these lifestyle choices by supporting metabolic health and contributing to a sense of satiety.

SAFETY CONSIDERATIONS

While licorice root is generally considered safe for most individuals when consumed in moderation, there are considerations to keep in mind. The primary concern is associated with glycyrrhizin, which can lead to an increase in blood pressure and potassium loss when consumed in excess. Individuals with hypertension, cardiovascular issues, or conditions that may be exacerbated by potassium depletion should exercise caution and consult with healthcare professionals before incorporating licorice root into their routine.

It's essential to choose deglycyrrhizinated licorice (DGL) products when aiming to avoid the potential side effects of glycyrrhizin. DGL products have undergone processing to remove or reduce glycyrrhizin, making them a safer option for long-term use.

FORSKOLIN

INTRODUCTION

Within the expansive world of herbal remedies, Forskolin (Coleus forskohlii) stands out as a powerful and captivating ally, renowned for its potential in aiding weight management. Derived from the roots of the Coleus forskohlii plant, forskolin has gained attention for its potential benefits in supporting fat metabolism and weight loss. Originating from traditional Ayurvedic medicine, this herbal compound has captured the attention of researchers and individuals alike. In this extensive exploration, we delve into the botanical foundations, active compounds, scientific research, and holistic integration of forskolin, uncovering its potential as a natural ally in the fight against obesity.

BOTANICAL FOUNDATIONS

Coleus forskohlii, a member of the mint family, is a perennial herb native to subtropical regions of Asia and Africa. The plant's roots are the source of forskolin, the bioactive compound that has become the focus of research into its potential health benefits. Traditionally, Coleus forskohlii has been utilized in Ayurvedic medicine for various purposes, including digestive and respiratory support. The plant's adaptability and resilience in diverse climates have contributed to its historical significance and its journey into modern herbal practices.

ACTIVE COMPOUNDS AND MECHANISMS OF ACTION

The key active compound in Coleus forskohlii is forskolin, a diterpene that acts by activating the enzyme adenylate cyclase. Adenylate cyclase is a crucial component in cellular signaling pathways that regulate the production of cyclic adenosine monophosphate (cAMP). Elevated cAMP levels influence various cellular functions, including the activation of protein kinase A (PKA), which, in turn, stimulates lipolysis – the breakdown of fats.

Forskolin's mechanism of action in promoting weight management revolves around its ability to enhance the cAMP-PKA pathway, which plays a role in the mobilization of stored fats. This process is believed to contribute to increased thermogenesis and the utilization of fats as a source of energy.

PREPARATION AND USAGE

Forskolin is commonly available in supplement form, often as capsules containing a standardized extract of Coleus forskohlii. The standardized extract ensures a consistent concentration of forskolin, typically ranging from 10% to 20%.

The recommended dosage of forskolin supplements can vary, and it is essential to follow product-specific guidelines or consult with healthcare professionals for personalized recommendations. It's crucial to choose high-quality supplements from reputable sources to ensure potency and safety.

HOLISTIC INTEGRATION INTO A HEALTHFUL LIFESTYLE

While forskolin holds promise as a herbal remedy for weight management, its potential unfolds most effectively within the context of a comprehensive approach to well-being. Forskolin should be viewed as a supportive element rather than a standalone solution in the journey towards weight wellness.

A balanced and nutrient-dense diet, regular physical activity, and mindful lifestyle choices remain fundamental to effective weight management. Forskolin's potential benefits can be optimized when integrated into a holistic framework that prioritizes overall health and well-being.

SAFETY CONSIDERATIONS

While forskolin is generally considered safe for most individuals when used as directed, there are considerations to be aware of. As with any herbal supplement, potential side effects and interactions with medications should be taken into account.

Common side effects of forskolin supplementation may include digestive issues such as diarrhea or nausea. Individuals with pre-existing medical conditions, especially cardiovascular issues, should exercise caution and consult with healthcare professionals before using forskolin.

Pregnant or breastfeeding individuals, as well as those with bleeding disorders or taking anticoagulant medications, should avoid forskolin due to its potential effects on blood clotting.

GUGGUL

INTRODUCTION

Guggul, a plant known as Commiphora wightii, has long been respected for its potential to help with a range of health issues, such as obesity. Hailing from the arid regions of India, Bangladesh, and Pakistan, Guggul boasts a rich heritage firmly entrenched in traditional Ayurvedic medicine. The resin derived from the Guggul tree has been highly valued in Ayurvedic practices for many years due to its potential benefits in promoting weight management. Through this in-depth exploration, we delve into the botanical foundations, active compounds, scientific research, and holistic integration of Guggul, uncovering its potential as a natural ally in the fight against obesity.

BOTANICAL FOUNDATIONS

Guggul, scientifically known as Commiphora wightii, is a small, thorny tree native to the Indian subcontinent. The resin extracted from the tree's bark, commonly referred to as Guggul or Indian Bdellium, is a central component in traditional Ayurvedic medicine. Guggul has a rich historical and cultural significance, with references to its use dating back to ancient Ayurvedic texts.

The Guggul tree thrives in arid and semi-arid regions, reflecting its resilience and adaptability. Its botanical foundations lie in the resinous exudate, which is obtained by making incisions in the bark. This resin undergoes processing to produce Guggul extract, a key ingredient in traditional Ayurvedic formulations.

ACTIVE COMPOUNDS AND MECHANISMS OF ACTION

The therapeutic potential of Guggul is attributed to its diverse array of bioactive compounds, with guggulsterones being the primary active constituents. Guggulsterones are plant sterols that exhibit a range of pharmacological actions, including anti-inflammatory and lipid-lowering effects.

One of the key mechanisms of action attributed to Guggul in the context of obesity management is its impact on lipid metabolism. Guggulsterones are believed to activate the farnesoid X receptor (FXR) and the peroxisome proliferator-activated receptor alpha (PPAR-alpha), both of which play essential roles in lipid regulation and metabolism.

PREPARATION AND USAGE

Guggul is commonly available in various forms, including Guggul extract, Guggul capsules, and Guggul powder. The standardized Guggul extract ensures a consistent concentration of guggulsterones, the bioactive compounds responsible for its potential health benefits.

The recommended dosage of Guggul supplements can vary, and it is essential to follow product-specific guidelines or consult with healthcare professionals for personalized recommendations. Guggul can be used as a standalone supplement or as part of Ayurvedic formulations targeting weight management.

HOLISTIC INTEGRATION INTO A HEALTHFUL LIFESTYLE

While Guggul holds promise as an herbal remedy for obesity, its potential benefits unfold most effectively within the context of a comprehensive approach to well-being. Guggul should be viewed as a supportive element in the journey towards weight wellness, complementing other healthful practices.

A balanced and nutrient-dense diet, regular physical activity, and mindful lifestyle choices remain foundational to effective weight management. Guggul's potential benefits can be optimized when integrated into a holistic framework that prioritizes overall health and well-being.

GINSENG

INTRODUCTION

Ginseng (Panax ginseng), a highly respected and ancient herb, is renowned for its adaptogenic qualities and potential to enhance overall health and wellness. With its roots in the mountainous regions of East Asia, Ginseng has made a lasting impact on the world of herbal medicine, transcending cultural and traditional boundaries. Although commonly linked to increased energy and overall well being, Ginseng has also been studied for its potential impact on weight management. Through a thorough examination, we explore the intricate world of botanicals, the compounds they contain, the scientific studies conducted, and the holistic approach to incorporating Ginseng. This reveals its potential as a natural ally in the fight against obesity.

BOTANICAL INTRICACIES

Ginseng, a member of the Araliaceae family, is a perennial herb with fleshy roots that is native to the cool, shaded forests of Eastern Asia, including China and Korea. The botanical name, Panax, is derived from the Greek words "pan," meaning all, and "axos," meaning cure, highlighting the esteemed reputation Ginseng has held throughout history.

There are various species of Ginseng, with Panax ginseng, Panax quinquefolius (American Ginseng), and Panax notoginseng being the most well-known. Panax ginseng, commonly referred to as Asian or Korean Ginseng, is the most widely studied and utilized in traditional herbal practices.

ACTIVE COMPOUNDS AND ADAPTOGENIC PROPERTIES

Ginseng's therapeutic properties are attributed to a complex interplay of bioactive compounds, most notably ginsenosides, which are triterpene saponins. These ginsenosides are considered the primary contributors to Ginseng's adaptogenic effects, aiding the body in adapting to various stressors and promoting balance.

The adaptogenic properties of Ginseng extend beyond stress response to include potential benefits for metabolism and energy regulation. While the specific mechanisms are intricate and multifaceted, ginsenosides are believed to interact with various signaling pathways, modulating the body's responses to stress and influencing metabolic processes.

PREPARATION AND CULINARY APPLICATIONS

Ginseng is available in various forms, including Ginseng root, Ginseng extract, Ginseng tea, and Ginseng supplements. The root, often dried and processed, can be used in traditional herbal formulations or brewed as a tea. Ginseng supplements, available in capsule or liquid form, offer a convenient option for those seeking standardized dosages of Ginseng's bioactive compounds.

Culinary applications of Ginseng are diverse, with Ginseng-infused dishes and beverages being a common practice in traditional Asian cuisine. Ginseng chicken soup, Ginseng tea, and Ginseng-infused desserts showcase the versatility of this revered herb in culinary creations.

HOLISTIC INTEGRATION INTO A HEALTHFUL LIFESTYLE

Ginseng's potential as an herbal remedy for obesity unfolds most effectively when viewed as part of a comprehensive strategy for well-being. While scientific findings provide valuable insights, Ginseng is not a standalone solution. Rather, it thrives in synergy with other healthful practices.

A balanced and nutrient-dense diet, regular physical activity, and mindful eating practices remain foundational to effective weight management. Ginseng, with its adaptogenic and potential metabolism-modulating effects, can complement these lifestyle choices by supporting the body's natural processes.

SAFETY CONSIDERATIONS

Ginseng is generally considered safe for most individuals when used as directed. However, certain considerations should be taken into account. Ginseng may interact with certain medications, including anticoagulants, antiplatelet drugs, and antidiabetic medications. Individuals with existing medical conditions or those taking medications should consult with healthcare professionals before incorporating Ginseng into their routine.

Additionally, excessive consumption of Ginseng may lead to side effects such as insomnia, increased heart rate, and digestive issues. It's crucial to follow recommended dosage guidelines and be mindful of individual responses.

PSYLLIUM

INTRODUCTION

Psyllium (Plantago ovata) is a remarkable source of dietary fiber that is highly regarded for its potential benefits in supporting digestive health and weight management. Hailing from the Mediterranean region, Psyllium has made its mark in both ancient healing traditions and modern wellness regimens. Thanks to its high soluble fiber content and its ability to support healthy digestion, Psyllium has become increasingly popular as a natural aid in managing weight. Through a thorough examination, we explore the botanical foundations, active compounds, scientific research, and holistic integration of Psyllium, uncovering its potential as a herbal remedy for weight wellness.

BOTANICAL FOUNDATIONS

Psyllium, derived from the seeds of Plantago ovata, is a herbaceous plant that belongs to the Plantaginaceae family. Native to regions in the Mediterranean, Psyllium has a long history of use in traditional medicine, particularly in Ayurveda. The plant produces tiny seeds encased in husks, and it is from these seeds that Psyllium husk, a rich source of soluble fiber, is obtained.

The adaptability of Plantago ovata is evident in its ability to thrive in various climates, making it a versatile and resilient botanical resource. The seeds, once processed into Psyllium husk or powder, become a valuable dietary supplement with a spectrum of potential health benefits.

ACTIVE COMPOUNDS AND SOLUBLE FIBER

The primary active compound in Psyllium responsible for its therapeutic properties is its high content of soluble fiber. Psyllium husk consists mainly of hemicellulose, a complex carbohydrate that forms a gel-like substance when mixed with water. This unique property of Psyllium makes it an exceptional source of soluble fiber, distinguishing it from other dietary fibers.

Soluble fiber, as opposed to insoluble fiber, dissolves in water to form a viscous gel. This gel-like consistency contributes to Psyllium's ability to absorb water, providing a gentle bulking effect in the digestive tract. The soluble fiber in Psyllium is composed of various polysaccharides, including arabinoxylan and xyloglucan, which contribute to its functional and health-promoting characteristics.

PREPARATION AND CULINARY APPLICATIONS

Psyllium is commonly available in various forms, including Psyllium husk, Psyllium powder, and Psyllium supplements. The husk or powder can be mixed with water, juice, or added to smoothies, providing a convenient and versatile way to incorporate Psyllium into daily dietary routines.

In culinary applications, Psyllium can be added to recipes to enhance their fiber content. It can be used as a binding or thickening agent in baking, particularly in gluten-free recipes. Psyllium's ability to absorb water and create a gel-like consistency makes it a valuable ingredient in recipes for bread, muffins, pancakes, and other baked goods.

HOLISTIC INTEGRATION INTO A HEALTHFUL LIFESTYLE

The integration of Psyllium into a healthful lifestyle extends beyond its potential benefits for weight management. Psyllium's soluble fiber content aligns with broader principles of digestive health and overall well-being.

A balanced and nutrient-dense diet, regular physical activity, and mindful eating practices remain fundamental to effective weight management. Psyllium, with its ability to promote satiety, support digestive regularity, and contribute to overall gut health, can be a valuable addition to a holistic approach to well-being.

SAFETY CONSIDERATIONS

Psyllium is generally considered safe for most individuals when used as directed. However, there are important considerations to ensure its safe and effective usage.

It is crucial to start with small amounts of Psyllium and gradually increase the intake while ensuring an adequate water intake. Psyllium absorbs water, and insufficient fluid intake may lead to potential issues such as bloating or constipation.

Individuals with certain medical conditions, such as gastrointestinal disorders or difficulty swallowing, should consult with healthcare professionals before using Psyllium. Additionally, it is advisable to take Psyllium away from medications, as it may interfere with their absorption.

BLACK PEPPER

INTRODUCTION

Black Pepper (Piper nigrum) is a versatile and powerful ingredient, known for its culinary versatility and potential positive effects on health. Hailing from the verdant hills of the Indian subcontinent, Black Pepper has journeyed across lands, blessing culinary creations and traditional remedies alike. Black Pepper is not just a spice enhancer, but also contains a variety of bioactive compounds that have caught the interest of scientists, particularly in relation to weight management. Join us on a journey as we delve into the fascinating world of Black Pepper, uncovering its botanical secrets, powerful compounds, extensive scientific studies, and its role in promoting holistic well-being.

BOTANICAL INTRICACIES

Black Pepper, belonging to the Piperaceae family, is a flowering vine cultivated for its fruit, which is commonly dried and used as a spice. Native to the Western Ghats of India, Black Pepper has been a prized commodity throughout history, influencing trade routes and culinary traditions.

The Piper nigrum vine bears clusters of small, round fruits known as peppercorns. The peppercorns undergo various processing methods to produce different forms of Black Pepper, such as black, white, and green pepper. Each variant offers a distinct flavor profile, with black pepper being the most commonly used.

The spicy kick of Black Pepper comes from the presence of piperine, a bioactive compound that contributes not only to its taste but also to its potential health-promoting properties.

ACTIVE COMPOUNDS AND PIPERINE

The primary bioactive compound in Black Pepper responsible for its therapeutic properties is piperine. Piperine is an alkaloid that gives Black Pepper its characteristic pungency and has been studied for various potential health benefits.

Beyond its role in enhancing flavor, piperine is known for its bioavailability-enhancing properties. It inhibits the activity of enzymes that participate in drug metabolism, leading to increased absorption of certain nutrients and compounds.

Piperine has also been explored for its potential impact on metabolism and weight management. Studies suggest that piperine may influence thermogenesis, the process by which the body generates heat and burns calories. Additionally, it may modulate lipid metabolism and adipocyte differentiation, contributing to its potential role in weight regulation.

PREPARATION AND CULINARY APPLICATIONS

Black Pepper is a versatile spice used in various culinary applications, adding depth and complexity to dishes. Its pungent flavor makes it a staple in kitchens worldwide, enhancing the taste of savory and even some sweet preparations.

In culinary applications, Black Pepper is often used in both its whole form and ground form. Whole peppercorns can be crushed or ground to release their flavors, while ground pepper offers convenience and ease of incorporation into recipes.

HOLISTIC INTEGRATION INTO A HEALTHFUL LIFESTYLE

The integration of Black Pepper into a healthful lifestyle extends beyond its potential benefits for weight management. While scientific findings provide valuable insights, Black Pepper is not a standalone solution. Instead, it complements other healthful practices in the journey towards overall well-being.

A balanced and nutrient-dense diet, regular physical activity, and mindful eating practices remain fundamental to effective weight management. Black Pepper, with its potential impact on metabolism, thermogenesis, and appetite regulation, can be a flavorful addition to dishes that support a holistic approach to well-being.

SAFETY CONSIDERATIONS

Black Pepper is generally considered safe for most individuals when used in culinary amounts. However, it's essential to note that excessive consumption of Black Pepper may lead to potential side effects, including gastrointestinal irritation.

Individuals with certain medical conditions, such as gastroesophageal reflux disease (GERD) or peptic ulcers, may need to moderate their intake of spicy foods, including Black Pepper, to avoid exacerbating symptoms.

Additionally, those with allergies to Piperaceae family plants should exercise caution and consult with healthcare professionals if considering Black Pepper supplements.

MUSTARD SEED

INTRODUCTION

Mustard Seed (Brassica juncea) is a small but mighty ingredient that is highly regarded for its culinary uses and potential health advantages. With its roots in the cruciferous family, Mustard Seed boasts a fascinating past that encompasses a wide range of culinary traditions and ancient healing methods. In addition to being a common spice, Mustard Seed contains bioactive compounds that have caught the attention of scientists due to their potential impact on weight management. Through a thorough examination, we explore the intricate world of Mustard Seed, uncovering its potential as a herbal remedy in combating obesity. We delve into its botanical properties, active compounds, scientific studies, and how it can be integrated into a holistic approach.

BOTANICAL INTRICACIES

Mustard Seed, derived from the Brassica juncea plant, belongs to the Brassicaceae family, which includes other cruciferous vegetables such as broccoli, cabbage, and kale. Native to regions of Asia, Mustard Seed has been cultivated for centuries, and its tiny seeds have become a staple in various cuisines worldwide.

The Brassica juncea plant produces small, round seeds that vary in color, ranging from yellow to brown. These seeds are rich in phytochemicals, including glucosinolates, which contribute to Mustard Seed's distinctive flavor and potential health benefits.

Mustard seeds can be processed to produce mustard oil, a culinary ingredient in some cultures, or ground into a powder for use as a spice. In traditional medicine, Mustard Seed has been recognized for its diverse applications, from digestive aid to respiratory support.

ACTIVE COMPOUNDS AND GLUCOSINOLATES

The primary bioactive compounds in Mustard Seed are glucosinolates, sulfur-containing compounds that are characteristic of cruciferous vegetables. These compounds are known for their potential health-promoting properties and have been studied for various therapeutic benefits.

Upon crushing or chewing, glucosinolates are enzymatically broken down into biologically active compounds, such as isothiocyanates, which are responsible for the pungent flavor and potential health effects of Mustard Seed.

Research has suggested that glucosinolates and their breakdown products may exert antioxidant, anti-inflammatory, and anti-cancer effects. Additionally, these compounds may play a role in metabolic processes, making Mustard Seed an intriguing subject for exploration in the context of weight management.

PREPARATION AND CULINARY APPLICATIONS

Mustard Seed is a versatile spice used in various culinary applications, adding depth and heat to dishes. Its unique flavor profile makes it a popular choice in spice blends, condiments, and pickles.

In culinary applications, Mustard Seed can be used in various forms, including whole seeds, ground powder, or prepared mustard paste. Whole seeds can be added to pickles or incorporated into spice blends, while ground Mustard Seed is a key ingredient in mustard sauce and spreads.

Beyond its role as a spice, Mustard Seed can also be incorporated into various recipes to impart its distinct flavor and potential health benefits. It pairs well with meats, vegetables, and marinades, offering a flavorful addition to a wide range of dishes.

HOLISTIC INTEGRATION INTO A HEALTHFUL LIFESTYLE

The integration of Mustard Seed into a healthful lifestyle extends beyond its potential benefits for weight management. While scientific findings provide valuable insights, Mustard Seed is not a standalone solution. Instead, it complements other healthful practices in the journey towards overall well-being.

A balanced and nutrient-dense diet, regular physical activity, and mindful eating practices remain fundamental to effective weight management. Mustard Seed, with its potential impact on metabolism, adipogenesis, and appetite regulation, can be a flavorful addition to dishes that support a holistic approach to well-being.

SAFETY CONSIDERATIONS

Mustard Seed is generally considered safe for most individuals when used in culinary amounts. However, it's essential to note that excessive consumption of Mustard Seed or its products may lead to potential side effects, including gastrointestinal irritation.

Individuals with certain medical conditions, such as gastroesophageal reflux disease (GERD) or sensitivity to spicy foods, may need to moderate their intake of Mustard Seed to avoid exacerbating symptoms.

Additionally, pregnant or breastfeeding individuals should consult with healthcare professionals before incorporating Mustard Seed supplements into their routine.

FENNEL

INTRODUCTION

Fennel (Foeniculum vulgare), known for its culinary versatility and potential health benefits, is a gentle yet powerful herb that has gained recognition. Hailing from the Mediterranean region, Fennel has become a staple in cuisines and natural remedies worldwide. In addition to being a delicious herb, Fennel contains bioactive compounds that have caught the attention of scientists due to their potential impact on weight management. Through a thorough examination, we explore the intricate world of Fennel, examining its active compounds, scientific studies, and its role as a holistic remedy in combating obesity.

BOTANICAL INTRICACIES

Fennel, belonging to the Apiaceae family, is a flowering herb known for its feathery leaves and aromatic seeds. Native to the Mediterranean region, Fennel has a rich history dating back to ancient times, where it found applications in culinary and medicinal practices.

The Foeniculum vulgare plant produces umbels of small yellow flowers and green, thread-like leaves. The seeds, commonly referred to as Fennel seeds, are the primary part used for both culinary and medicinal purposes. Fennel's distinct flavor, reminiscent of licorice, imparts a unique taste to dishes and makes it a popular addition to various cuisines.

ACTIVE COMPOUNDS AND PHYTOCHEMICALS

The therapeutic properties of Fennel are attributed to a diverse array of bioactive compounds and phytochemicals present in its seeds and leaves. These include essential oils, flavonoids, phenolic compounds, and anethole, a major component contributing to Fennel's characteristic flavor.

Anethole, a compound with a molecular structure similar to estrogen, has been studied for its potential health benefits. It exhibits antioxidant, anti-inflammatory, and antimicrobial properties, and research suggests that it may play a role in various physiological processes.

Fennel seeds also contain fiber, which contributes to their potential benefits for digestion and satiety. The fiber content may play a role in supporting digestive health and promoting a feeling of fullness, factors that can be relevant in the context of weight management.

PREPARATION AND CULINARY APPLICATIONS

Fennel is a versatile herb that lends itself to various culinary applications, contributing its unique flavor profile to dishes ranging from salads to desserts. The entire plant, including the bulb, leaves, and seeds, is utilized in different ways in culinary traditions around the world.

Fennel seeds, with their aromatic and slightly sweet taste, are often used as a spice and flavoring agent. They can be added to both sweet and savory dishes, including baked goods, soups, stews, and pickles. In Indian cuisine, Fennel seeds are commonly consumed as a post-meal digestive aid.

The bulb of the Fennel plant has a crisp texture and a mild, licorice-like flavor. It can be sliced and added to salads, roasted as a side dish, or used in soups and sautés. Fennel leaves, also known as fronds, can be used as a garnish or incorporated into salads and dressings.

HOLISTIC INTEGRATION INTO A HEALTHFUL LIFESTYLE

The integration of Fennel into a healthful lifestyle extends beyond its potential benefits for weight management. While scientific findings provide valuable insights, Fennel is not a standalone solution. Instead, it complements other healthful practices in the journey towards overall well-being.

A balanced and nutrient-dense diet, regular physical activity, and mindful eating practices remain fundamental to effective weight management. Fennel, with its potential impact on appetite regulation, metabolism, and inflammation, can be a flavorful addition to dishes that support a holistic approach to well-being.

SAFETY CONSIDERATIONS

Fennel is generally considered safe for most individuals when consumed in culinary amounts. However, certain considerations should be taken into account to ensure its safe and effective usage.

Individuals who are allergic to celery, carrots, or other plants in the Apiaceae family may be more prone to allergic reactions to Fennel. It's advisable to exercise caution and seek medical advice if allergic reactions occur.

Pregnant or breastfeeding individuals should consult with healthcare professionals before using Fennel supplements, as the safety of higher doses during pregnancy is not well-established.

CUMIN

INTRODUCTION

Cumin (Cuminum cyminum), known for its delightful aroma and versatile uses in the kitchen, is highly regarded for its potential positive effects on health. Hailing from the Mediterranean and now grown all over the world, Cumin has become an integral part of various culinary traditions and alternative healthcare methods. Scientific interest has been piqued by the bioactive compounds found in Cumin, which go beyond its traditional use as a spice. These compounds have shown potential in the realm of weight management. Join us on a deep dive into the world of Cumin, where we explore its botanical complexities, active compounds, scientific studies, and its role in holistic approaches to achieving weight wellness.

BOTANICAL INTRICACIES

Cumin, belonging to the Apiaceae family, is a flowering plant known for its aromatic seeds. Native to regions stretching from the eastern Mediterranean to India, Cumin has been cultivated for thousands of years, leaving its aromatic imprint on cuisines spanning continents.

The Cuminum cyminum plant produces small, elongated seeds that boast a distinctive warm and earthy flavor. The seeds are the primary part used for culinary and medicinal purposes. Ground Cumin is a staple spice in various spice blends, while whole seeds are often toasted or used in cooking to impart a rich and nutty aroma.

ACTIVE COMPOUNDS AND PHYTOCHEMICALS

The therapeutic properties of Cumin are attributed to a range of bioactive compounds and phytochemicals present in its seeds. These include essential oils, cuminaldehyde, flavonoids, and various antioxidants that contribute to Cumin's flavor profile and potential health benefits.

Cuminaldehyde, a major component of Cumin essential oil, has demonstrated antioxidant and anti-inflammatory properties in scientific studies. These properties are of particular interest in the context of obesity, where chronic inflammation is often associated with adipose tissue dysfunction.

Cumin is also a rich source of flavonoids, which are known for their antioxidant and anti-inflammatory effects. The combination of these bioactive compounds positions Cumin as a spice with potential health-promoting properties beyond its culinary appeal.

PREPARATION AND CULINARY APPLICATIONS

Cumin is a versatile spice that plays a central role in the culinary traditions of many cultures. Its warm and earthy flavor makes it a popular addition to a wide range of dishes, from soups and stews to spice blends and roasted vegetables.

In culinary applications, Cumin can be used in both its whole seed and ground forms. Whole seeds are often toasted to enhance their flavor before being added to dishes. Ground Cumin is a key ingredient in spice mixes such as curry powder and is used to season meats, vegetables, and legumes.

The aromatic qualities of Cumin contribute not only to its taste but also to its ability to enhance the overall sensory experience of a dish. Its warm and slightly nutty notes make it a favorite in both savory and sweet recipes, showcasing its versatility in the kitchen.

HOLISTIC INTEGRATION INTO A HEALTHFUL LIFESTYLE

The integration of Cumin into a healthful lifestyle extends beyond its potential benefits for weight management. While scientific findings provide valuable insights, Cumin is not a standalone solution. Instead, it complements other healthful practices in the journey towards overall well-being.

A balanced and nutrient-dense diet, regular physical activity, and mindful eating practices remain fundamental to effective weight management. Cumin, with its potential impact on appetite regulation, metabolic parameters, and inflammation, can be a flavorful addition to dishes that support a holistic approach to well-being.

SAFETY CONSIDERATIONS

Cumin is generally considered safe for most individuals when consumed in culinary amounts. However, certain considerations should be taken into account to ensure its safe and effective usage.

Individuals who are allergic to plants in the Apiaceae family, such as celery or fennel, may be more prone to allergic reactions to Cumin. It's advisable to exercise caution and seek medical advice if allergic reactions occur.

Additionally, pregnant or breastfeeding individuals should consult with healthcare professionals before using Cumin supplements, as the safety of higher doses during pregnancy is not well-established.

CARDAMOM

INTRODUCTION

In the rich tapestry of herbal remedies, Cardamom (Elettaria cardamomum) emerges as a fragrant and versatile ally, celebrated for its culinary allure and potential health benefits. Originating from the lush landscapes of the Indian subcontinent, Cardamom has traversed centuries to become a staple in global cuisines and traditional medicine practices. Beyond its role as a spice, Cardamom harbors bioactive compounds that have captured scientific attention, particularly in the realm of weight management. In this comprehensive exploration, we navigate through the botanical intricacies, active compounds, scientific research, and holistic integration of Cardamom, unraveling its fragrant trail in the battle against obesity.

BOTANICAL INTRICACIES

Cardamom, a member of the Zingiberaceae family, is a perennial herb with rhizomatous roots. Native to the Western Ghats of India, Cardamom is renowned for its distinct and captivating flavor profile. The Elettaria cardamomum plant produces small, green pods containing aromatic seeds. These seeds, often referred to as Cardamom seeds, are the primary part used for culinary and medicinal purposes.

The cultivation of Cardamom has expanded beyond its native regions, with Guatemala, India, and Sri Lanka being major producers. The plant's adaptability and resilience contribute to its widespread availability and use in various cultural and culinary traditions.

ACTIVE COMPOUNDS AND ESSENTIAL OILS

The therapeutic properties of Cardamom are attributed to a rich array of bioactive compounds, including essential oils, terpenes, and antioxidants. These compounds contribute not only to Cardamom's distinctive aroma and flavor but also to its potential health-promoting effects.

One of the key components in Cardamom essential oil is 1,8-cineole, also known as eucalyptol. This compound possesses anti-inflammatory and antioxidant properties, making it a valuable contributor to Cardamom's potential health benefits.

Additionally, Cardamom contains terpenes like limonene and pinene, which contribute to its aromatic profile and have been studied for their potential therapeutic effects. Limonene, for example, is known for its anti-inflammatory and anti-cancer properties.

PREPARATION AND CULINARY APPLICATIONS

Cardamom is a versatile spice that adds a unique and aromatic dimension to a wide range of culinary creations. Its warm and slightly citrusy flavor makes it a prized ingredient in both sweet and savory dishes.

In culinary applications, Cardamom can be used in various forms, including whole pods, seeds, or ground powder. Whole pods are often added to rice dishes, stews, and desserts, infusing the dish with their distinct aroma during cooking. Ground Cardamom is a common addition to baked goods, beverages, and spice blends.

Cardamom's versatility extends to its use in traditional beverages, such as chai tea. In some cultures, Cardamom is also used to flavor coffee or incorporated into refreshing beverages.

HOLISTIC INTEGRATION INTO A HEALTHFUL LIFESTYLE

The integration of Cardamom into a healthful lifestyle extends beyond its potential benefits for weight management. While scientific findings provide valuable insights, Cardamom is not a standalone solution. Instead, it complements other healthful practices in the journey towards overall well-being.

A balanced and nutrient-dense diet, regular physical activity, and mindful eating practices remain fundamental to effective weight management. Cardamom, with its potential impact on metabolic parameters, appetite regulation, and inflammation, can be a flavorful addition to dishes that support a holistic approach to well-being.

SAFETY CONSIDERATIONS

Cardamom is generally considered safe for most individuals when consumed in culinary amounts. However, certain considerations should be taken into account to ensure its safe and effective usage.

Individuals who are allergic to plants in the Zingiberaceae family, such as ginger or turmeric, may be more prone to allergic reactions to Cardamom. It's advisable to exercise caution and seek medical advice if allergic reactions occur.

Additionally, pregnant or breastfeeding individuals should consult with healthcare professionals before using Cardamom supplements, as the safety of higher doses during pregnancy is not well-established.

BLACK CUMIN SEED

INTRODUCTION

In the vast realm of herbal remedies, Black Cumin Seed (Nigella sativa) emerges as a hidden gem, celebrated for its historical significance and potential health benefits. Originating from the Mediterranean region and cultivated in various parts of the world, Black Cumin Seed has been revered for centuries for its culinary and medicinal properties. Beyond its role as a spice, Black Cumin Seed harbors bioactive compounds that have sparked scientific interest, particularly in the context of weight management. In this comprehensive exploration, we navigate through the botanical intricacies, active compounds, scientific research, and holistic integration of Black Cumin Seed, uncovering its potential as a herbal remedy in the fight against obesity.

BOTANICAL INTRICACIES

Black Cumin Seed, also known as Nigella sativa or Kalonji, belongs to the Ranunculaceae family. The plant is characterized by delicate, feathery leaves and white or pale blue flowers. The small, crescent-shaped seeds of the Nigella sativa plant are the primary part used for both culinary and medicinal purposes.

Native to the Mediterranean region, Black Cumin Seed has a rich history that spans ancient civilizations, including its mention in ancient Egyptian texts and Islamic traditions. The versatility of Black Cumin Seed extends to its culinary applications, where it is often used as a spice in various cuisines.

ACTIVE COMPOUNDS AND PHYTOCHEMICALS

The therapeutic properties of Black Cumin Seed are attributed to a diverse array of bioactive compounds and phytochemicals present in its seeds. These include thymoquinone, thymohydroquinone, dithymoquinone, and a range of antioxidants.

Thymoquinone, a major bioactive component of Black Cumin Seed, has garnered attention for its potential anti-inflammatory, antioxidant, and anti-cancer properties. Research has explored its impact on various physiological processes, making it a focal point in understanding the potential health benefits of Black Cumin Seed.

Antioxidants present in Black Cumin Seed contribute to its overall health-promoting effects. These antioxidants, including carotenoids and tocopherols, play a crucial role in neutralizing free radicals and protecting cells from oxidative stress.

PREPARATION AND CULINARY APPLICATIONS

Black Cumin Seed is a versatile spice that adds a distinctive flavor to a variety of dishes. Its slightly bitter, peppery taste makes it a unique addition to both savory and sweet recipes.

In culinary applications, Black Cumin Seed can be used in various forms, including whole seeds, ground powder, or as an oil. Whole seeds are often toasted to enhance their flavor before being added to dishes. Ground Black Cumin Seed can be incorporated into spice blends, marinades, and sauces.

Black Cumin Seed oil is also utilized in cooking and as a finishing oil for salads and other dishes. It adds a rich and nutty flavor, complementing the overall taste profile of a dish.

HOLISTIC INTEGRATION INTO A HEALTHFUL LIFESTYLE

The integration of Black Cumin Seed into a healthful lifestyle extends beyond its potential benefits for weight management. While scientific findings provide valuable insights, Black Cumin Seed is not a standalone solution. Instead, it complements other healthful practices in the journey towards overall well-being.

A balanced and nutrient-dense diet, regular physical activity, and mindful eating practices remain fundamental to effective weight management. Black Cumin Seed, with its potential impact on metabolism, appetite regulation, and inflammation, can be a flavorful addition to dishes that support a holistic approach to well-being.

SAFETY CONSIDERATIONS

Black Cumin Seed is generally considered safe for most individuals when consumed in culinary amounts. However, certain considerations should be taken into account to ensure its safe and effective usage.

Individuals who are allergic to plants in the Ranunculaceae family, such as buttercups or anemones, may be more prone to allergic reactions to Black Cumin Seed. It's advisable to exercise caution and seek medical advice if allergic reactions occur.

Additionally, pregnant or breastfeeding individuals should consult with healthcare professionals before using Black Cumin Seed supplements, as the safety of higher doses during pregnancy is not well-established.

TRIPHALA

INTRODUCTION

In the vast landscape of herbal remedies, Triphala stands as an ancient and revered elixir, celebrated for its holistic approach to well-being and potential health benefits. Originating from the traditional system of Ayurveda in India, Triphala has transcended centuries to become a cornerstone in natural health practices. Beyond its historical significance, Triphala has garnered attention for its potential contributions to weight management. In this comprehensive exploration, we delve into the botanical intricacies, active compounds, scientific research, and holistic integration of Triphala, unraveling its multifaceted role as a herbal remedy in the pursuit of weight wellness.

BOTANICAL INTRICACIES

Triphala, a Sanskrit compound meaning "three fruits," is a blend of three key fruits: Amalaki (Emblica officinalis), Bibhitaki (Terminalia bellirica), and Haritaki (Terminalia chebula). These fruits, each with unique properties, synergize to form a potent herbal concoction.

Amalaki, also known as Indian gooseberry, contributes its rich vitamin C content and antioxidant properties. Bibhitaki, derived from the Baheda tree, is esteemed for its astringent qualities. Haritaki, sourced from the Harada tree, is revered for its rejuvenating and digestive benefits. The combination of these three fruits creates a harmonious herbal formula that has been cherished for centuries.

ACTIVE COMPOUNDS AND SYNERGISTIC EFFECTS

The therapeutic properties of Triphala stem from the diverse array of bioactive compounds present in its constituent fruits. These include tannins, polyphenols, flavonoids, vitamins, and essential oils. The synergistic effects of these compounds contribute to Triphala's potential health-promoting properties.

Tannins, known for their astringent properties, play a role in supporting digestive health. Polyphenols, with their antioxidant effects, contribute to cellular protection from oxidative stress. Flavonoids, recognized for their anti-inflammatory properties, enhance Triphala's overall impact on well-being.

The synergistic combination of Amalaki, Bibhitaki, and Haritaki creates a balanced herbal formulation. Amalaki's vitamin C content complements Bibhitaki's astringency and Haritaki's rejuvenating qualities. This synergy is a hallmark of Ayurvedic principles, where the combination of herbs is believed to enhance their individual efficacy.

PREPARATION AND CULINARY APPLICATIONS

Triphala is traditionally prepared as a powdered herbal supplement, and its consumption is deeply rooted in Ayurvedic practices. The powder can be mixed with water, honey, or warm milk to create a tonic. Additionally, Triphala is available in capsule or tablet form for convenient consumption.

The traditional preparation involves combining equal parts of Amalaki, Bibhitaki, and Haritaki powders. The blend is then carefully mixed to ensure a balanced representation of each fruit. The resulting Triphala powder encapsulates the synergistic benefits of the three fruits.

While Triphala itself is not a culinary spice, its powdered form can be incorporated into recipes or consumed with warm water as a daily tonic. Some traditional recipes may include Triphala in herbal teas or Ayurvedic formulations designed to support overall health.

HOLISTIC INTEGRATION INTO A HEALTHFUL LIFESTYLE

The integration of Triphala into a healthful lifestyle extends beyond its potential benefits for weight management. In Ayurveda, the approach to well-being encompasses not only physical health but also mental and spiritual harmony.

Triphala is often recommended in Ayurvedic practices as part of a holistic regimen. Alongside dietary considerations, it is advised to cultivate mindful eating habits, engage in regular physical activity, and foster mental well-being. These practices align with the holistic principles of Ayurveda, which views health as a harmonious balance of various elements.

The adaptogenic qualities of Triphala contribute to its holistic benefits. Adaptogens are substances that help the body adapt to stressors, promoting overall resilience. In the context of weight management, the adaptogenic properties of Triphala may support the body's ability to respond to various stressors, both internal and external.

SAFETY CONSIDERATIONS

Triphala is generally considered safe for most individuals when consumed as directed. However, it's crucial to consider individual variations and potential interactions with existing health conditions or medications.

Pregnant or breastfeeding individuals should consult with healthcare professionals before using Triphala supplements, as the safety of higher doses during pregnancy is not well-established.

In some cases, mild digestive discomfort, such as bloating or loose stools, may occur initially. Adjusting the dosage or consulting with a healthcare provider can help address these concerns.

As with any herbal supplement, it's advisable to source Triphala from reputable sources to ensure product quality and purity.

HIBISCUS

INTRODUCTION

In the vast world of herbal remedies, Hibiscus emerges as a vibrant and aromatic contender, celebrated for its cultural significance and potential health benefits. With its showy blossoms and tart flavor, Hibiscus sabdariffa has captivated hearts around the globe. Beyond its ornamental beauty, Hibiscus harbors bioactive compounds that have piqued scientific curiosity, particularly in the realm of weight management. In this comprehensive exploration, we delve into the botanical intricacies, active compounds, scientific research, and holistic integration of Hibiscus, unfolding its petals in the battle against obesity.

BOTANICAL INTRICACIES

Hibiscus sabdariffa, commonly known as Roselle or Hibiscus, belongs to the Malvaceae family. This flowering plant is characterized by its vibrant red calyces, which are the fleshy structures that surround the seed pods. The calyces are commonly used in culinary and medicinal preparations.

Native to tropical regions, Hibiscus has found its way into various cultures and traditions, where it is valued for both its aesthetic appeal and potential health-promoting properties. The plant's adaptability and versatility have led to its cultivation in different parts of the world.

ACTIVE COMPOUNDS AND PHYTOCHEMICALS

The therapeutic properties of Hibiscus are attributed to a rich array of bioactive compounds and phytochemicals present in its calyces. These include anthocyanins, flavonoids, polyphenols, and organic acids.

Anthocyanins are responsible for the vibrant red hue of Hibiscus calyces and contribute to its antioxidant properties. These compounds have been studied for their potential in combating oxidative stress, a factor often associated with obesity-related complications.

Flavonoids, another group of compounds found in Hibiscus, have anti-inflammatory and cardiovascular benefits. Quercetin, one of the flavonoids present, has been studied for its potential in modulating metabolic processes and supporting overall health.

Polyphenols in Hibiscus contribute to its overall antioxidant capacity, protecting cells from damage caused by free radicals. Additionally, organic acids, such as hibiscus acid and citric acid, contribute to the tart flavor of Hibiscus and may play a role in its potential health benefits.

PREPARATION AND CULINARY APPLICATIONS

Hibiscus is commonly consumed as a floral infusion, creating a vibrant and tangy beverage known as Hibiscus tea or sorrel. The dried calyces are steeped in hot water, imparting their distinctive color and flavor to the infusion. Hibiscus tea can be enjoyed hot or cold and is often sweetened with natural sweeteners like honey or agave.

Apart from its use in beverages, Hibiscus can be incorporated into culinary creations. The dried calyces can be used in jams, jellies, and sauces, adding a unique tartness to the dishes. Additionally, Hibiscus is sometimes used as a flavoring agent in desserts, giving a floral and citrusy twist to recipes.

The versatility of Hibiscus extends to its use in spice blends and marinades, where it contributes both flavor and a visually appealing hue. The tart and slightly floral notes of Hibiscus make it a versatile ingredient that complements both sweet and savory dishes.

HOLISTIC INTEGRATION INTO A HEALTHFUL LIFESTYLE

The integration of Hibiscus into a healthful lifestyle extends beyond its potential benefits for weight management. In holistic wellness practices, Hibiscus is valued not only for its physiological effects but also for its sensory and ritualistic qualities.

Hibiscus tea, with its vibrant color and refreshing taste, can be incorporated into mindful moments and self-care rituals. Taking a moment to enjoy a cup of Hibiscus tea, whether in the morning or during a break, provides an opportunity to pause, savor, and engage in a calming sensory experience.

In Ayurveda, traditional Indian medicine, Hibiscus is sometimes recommended for its potential cooling properties. In this context, it may be used seasonally or in accordance with individual constitutions as part of a holistic approach to well-being.

The adaptogenic qualities of Hibiscus, seen in its ability to adapt to different culinary applications, resonate with the holistic concept of adaptability in well-being. Just as Hibiscus adapts its flavor to various dishes, individuals can adapt their lifestyle choices to support overall health and wellness.

SAFETY CONSIDERATIONS

Hibiscus tea is generally considered safe for most individuals when consumed in moderation. However, certain considerations should be taken into account to ensure its safe and effective usage.

Hibiscus tea may interact with certain medications, including antihypertensive drugs. Individuals taking medication for blood pressure should consult with healthcare professionals before incorporating hibiscus into their routine.

In some cases, excessive consumption of Hibiscus tea may lead to gastrointestinal discomfort. It's advisable to start with small amounts and monitor individual tolerance.

Pregnant or breastfeeding individuals should consult with healthcare professionals before consuming hibiscus tea, as its safety during pregnancy is not well-established.

The End